Good Morning . . . Let the Stress Begin

and other writings to encourage you
to publish your own stories

by

Phyllis Porter Dolislager

Dedication

To my husband, **Ronald Dolislager**

He's my best friend,

my favorite person in the whole world,

and a wonderful helpmate.

His servant's heart is seen not only by me,

but by all those who worked with him:

24 years at South America Mission,

one year at First Baptist Church of W. P. B.,

nine years at World Mission Centre/Live School.

I love you, Ron.

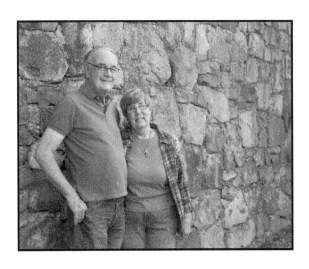

Preface

In an effort to showcase various subjects/topics that are appropriate for POD (Print on Demand) publishing or Internet publishing, I've put this book together. You'll find personal essays, poetry, excerpts from a personal memoir and a family memoir, and even a little humor.

You'll also find that there are a lot of writings that pertain to my post-polio. I've included them for those who also live with a chronic illness or disability, and for their caregivers.

It is my hope that you'll find some inspiration to write your own stories and to do your own publishing. I have used Xulon Press, Instant Publisher, iUniverse, and currently CreateSpace. Check them out, and you'll be on your way to an adventure.

Fulfil a dream. Amaze your family. Pass on your heritage. Share your thoughts. Be a published author. It can all become a reality.

And if you need help, contact me. I'm a writing consultant and have helped over 50+ people get their words in print. You could be the next one.

Contents

Good Morning . . . Let the Stress Begin

The events of 9/11, followed by the war in Afghanistan, the war in Iraq, more global turmoil and natural disasters, then the terrorist attacks in the U.S., and even local violence have thrown our entire nation into stress overload. We've become addicted to watching the news unfold on TV and online. Nationwide our stress levels haven't returned to their pre-9/11 levels. We've gotten used to it and haven't learned how to function without it.

We are constantly experiencing wild and confusing times. We've seen sniper shootings, kidnappings, school shootings, computer viruses that almost stopped the world's businesses, and the election that took 37 days in 2000. Through TV, newspapers, the Internet, imbedded reporters, and cell phones, we've been brought face to face with war and local violence.   That's stress producing, for sure.

Although it didn't make the headlines, August of 1999, I had my own stressful experience. I found myself in an ambulance, on a stretcher, being taken to the emergency room of our local hospital. 9-1-1 had been called because I was having chest pains and maybe a heart attack.

I remember lying on that stretcher as they carried me out from my office thinking, *I am going to die*. I was struggling to breathe. Two nurses began working on me.

Because of my family history, I stayed overnight and had a stress test the next day. There was a young man who administered my test, and he really impressed me. (I might as well confess right now, I am a Type "A" personality, and I wanted to hire him.) My staff needed someone just like him. So right there with all those tapes/monitors on my chest, I interviewed him.

"Are you a college graduate?" I asked. "Good. You're a Gator? Well, alright." (For those of you who don't know, that means he went to the University of Florida in Gainesville.) I returned to my room with his phone number!

It probably was no surprise to find out that I did not have a heart attack. My diagnosis was STRESS. (One author I read defined stress as: accelerated dying.)

I'll admit that I had known that my life was full of stress. And I'd even done something about it — I had planned a week at the beach, and fortunately that week started the day after I left the hospital.

I returned to my job of directing a teen pregnancy and STD (sexually transmitted diseases) prevention program. I purchased a sign and put it on the wall in my office. It read: "Good Morning…Let the Stress Begin".

I cut back to working four days a week. But I always checked my planner before I scheduled my day off. This really meant that I did five days of work in four. I followed this regiment for six months, and finally I knew if I was going to recapture my life and my health, I needed to resign.

How did I know that I had too much stress, you might ask? I had seen many lists of symptoms. I didn't have all of them, but I had way too many.

SYMPTOMS OF STRESS

Insomnia
I was such a Type A personality that I slept with a notepad and pencil on my nightstand. I'd wake up with an idea and write it down in case I wouldn't remember it in the morning.

Headaches
I was one of the best customers Advil ever had.

Fatigue
I'd come home and fall on the couch at night. I didn't even cook. I had Ron bring the food in!

Tense Shoulders
That's where we carry our worries.

Heartburn/ulcer
How many of us carry antacid with us?
I was popping them regularly.

Diarrhea or constipation
Yes.

Weight gain or lose
I put on 20 lbs.
(Spelled backwards, stressed is Desserts!)

Poor concentration
I'm an avid reader, but I wasn't reading books anymore, just magazines and the newspaper.

Increased use of alcohol or tobacco
One symptom I didn't have.

Stress sabotages our bodies — from our heads on down.
Remember the definition I gave earlier?
Accelerated dying.

CAUSES OF STRESS TODAY

1. **Super Woman or Super Man Syndrome**
"Be all that you can be," says the Army, and we all believe it. My Teen Pregnancy Prevention Program had become a state model. If the Department of Health in Tallahassee received questions about how to run a similar program, they'd send them to observe us. (And by the way, we did hire that young man I met and interviewed in the hospital!)

2. Accessibility

We're never alone.

We carry our phones with us all the time — to the dinner table, to meetings, even to church. E-mail lets us work anytime, anywhere, 24/7.

Cell phones reach us any place. I'm glad I have one, but other people and their phones annoy me: more stress!!

3. Busy Calendars

We wanted to have friends to dinner on a Friday night and had to schedule them five weeks out for our calendars to coincide. And we get together only once a year!

4. Analysis Overload[1]

Menus — can take ten minutes to read; even fast food chains give us many choices.

Cereal — there are over 100 choices

Soap — 249 kinds

Toothpaste — 250 kinds

Tennis shoes — can be so complicated to buy that you almost need to do research.

TV — my service gives me 200+ choices, and that's only a portion of what's available.

5. Consumer Orgy

Shopping makes us feel good, doesn't it?

How many **TV's** do we have in our homes?

How many of us have **clothes** overflowing into the guest room closet?

Do you have more than ten pair of **shoes** in your
    closet?
Duplicate **tools** in your garage?
Keeping up with "what's in" is stressful.

6. **Hurry Syndrome**
I was born into this stress producer. My best-selling
book, *Lessons Learned on the Farm*, is about growing up
on a dairy farm in the 50's and 60's. The working title
was "Our Clocks Were Set 10 Minutes Ahead," and they
were!

Today we use our DVR/X1 box to automatically fast-
forward over commercials. (This way we can watch a 30-
minute program in 22 minutes!)

We e-mail rather than write longhand letters—it's faster.

We send packages by Federal Express.
We use Sprint for telephone calls.
We use Quicken to manage our finances.
We diet with Slim Fast!

7. **Living away from family**
Having to travel long distances to see family and not
seeing them often is stressful. Our sons and their families
live in Arkansas and Tennessee. Most of our other
relatives are in Michigan and California. And for 30+
years, we lived in Florida. We missed that familial
support system a lot.

8. Traffic

We'd never even heard of road rage five years ago. Now they plant trees and flowers to calm us down — at least in South Florida, on I-95, they do. However, we have no proof that it's working.

9. Facing our own mortality

Realizing we're going to die someday and then what?

For me it wasn't 9/11, but facing the big Five-O. My own mortality suddenly hit me like a ton of bricks. I'd wake up in the middle of the night and literally jump out of bed saying to myself, "I'm still here, I'm living, I'm breathing."

All of a sudden, the thought of being somewhere else was so disconcerting, so strange, that even if it were heaven, I could hardly breathe. I'd get up and walk around and then go back to bed.

I also started to think, *I only have 20 years left to live*. (The Bible does say, *three score and ten*) *I probably won't see my grandchildren get married*, and on and on it went. This continued for two or three weeks. It was with me during the daylight hours, and it awakened me at night.

Until one day a Scripture verse popped up in front of my eyes. *For I know the plans that I have for you, declares the Lord, . . . plans to give you hope and a future.*
Jeremiah 29:11 (NIV)

God's Word to the rescue. I can't begin to tell you what a comfort that was to me. First of all, if God still had **plans** for me, I decided that I'd better not fret whether I had 20 years or 20 days to live. I needed to get on with my life and trust Him for the strength.

That scripture also said, *plans to give us a future and a hope.* Do you know what that "future and hope" are? Ultimately, they're eternal life!

Whatever your pain, whatever your problem, whatever your stress, Jesus Christ is the answer. Even if you fear death--Jesus conquered death when he rose from the dead on Easter morning 2,000 years ago.

Jesus and Jesus alone has the words of eternal life. Scripture says, *He* (Jesus) *swallowed up death for all time.* (Isaiah 25:8)

And our most favorite psalm, Psalm 23 says, *Even though I walk through the valley of the shadow of death, I will fear no evil, for You are with me.*   *(NKJV)*

**Having a relationship with Jesus Christ
is the biggest step toward
stress reduction you can take.**

It's encouraging to know that the American public has embraced faith as a stress reducer since 9-11. We never used to hear news people say, "Our thoughts and prayers are with you." And all of a sudden, it's OK to say "God," even on national TV.

The Parade Magazine, which many of us read in our Sunday newspaper, had this secondary headline in its March 23, 2003 issue: *Prayer and faith speeded recovery in illnesses ranging from depression, to stroke, to heart attack.* It went on to tell of studies, with funding from the National Institute of Health (NIH), by investigators at Johns Hopkins, the University of Pennsylvania, and Baptist Memorial Hospital in Memphis. "We are trying to see whether prayer has meaning to people that translates into biology and affects a disease process."

"Medical acceptance has grown along with solid scientific data on prayer's impact, says Dr. Dale Matthews of Georgetown University, author of *The Faith Factor.*" The article continues by quoting Dr. Matthews, "If prayer were available in pill form, no pharmacy could stock enough of it."

Another secondary headline reads: *Those who pray stay healthier and live longer than those who don't.* The article concludes by quoting Dr. Harold Koenig of Duke University's Center for the Study of Religion/Spirituality and Health. He says, "We now know enough, based on solid research, to say that prayer, much like exercise and diet, has a connection with better health."

Yes, stress did a number on me, but I wasn't about to let it become the "guest that came to dinner and stayed for the entire Olympics." Let me share some ideas that were helpful.

14 WAYS TO REDUCE YOUR STRESS

1. Exercise regularly
Take a walk, use exercise videos or join a gym — whatever works for you. And exercise your mind by playing games, doing crossword puzzles or my favorite, Sudoku.

2. Listen to music without words
Have it playing in your house. Who cares if they call it? "elevator music?" Elevators are a place where calmness is a *good* thing.

3. Learn to say the two-letter word, "NO."
Be brutally honest with yourself about what you can eliminate from your routine. Busyness is not a virtue.

4. Get lots of sunshine
Studies show that it's true: sunshine relieves depression. I know I thrived on the sunshine we have in South Florida. It sure beats those gray, days I remember in Michigan.

5. Talk to a trained counselor or clergy

Going to a counselor could be the best gift you ever give yourself. Inadvertently, I ended up talking to one for the first time. God put an experienced psychologist in my family doctor's office on the day that I had an appointment. He was extremely helpful. I would never hesitate to speak with one of my pastors or a counselor.

6. Laugh More

A 4-year old laughs every four minutes. They say that the average adult laughs 15 times a day. I found that I was an under-achiever in this category. I shared these stats with a friend who was also going through some stress. Later when we met for lunch, she said, "I came to do some laughing." Another time we got together with our husbands, and each one of us brought a joke to share.

Have you laughed today? It's very healthy; some call it "inner jogging". Read the comics in the newspaper. Buy a joke book or find some jokes online. Watch a comedy video.

7. Spend time with people you enjoy.

I consciously try to spend time with people who are uplifting. I don't need the negativity that some carry around and so liberally dispense.

8. **Change your value system.**
Here are three principles to remember:
      1. People are more important than things.
      2. People are more important than things,
      3. People are more important than things.

9. **Get a massage or sit in a hot tub.**
Give yourself permission to take the time (and expense) to do something for yourself. You're worth it.

10. **Keep a journal.**
I am a writer, but this was a new experience for me. Trust me. Putting it on paper is a wonderful release. The stress goes from your shoulders to the journal pages. And who knows, it might give our grandchildren or nieces and nephews something to read after we're gone.

11. **Make a doctor's appointment**.
Our bodies are the first victims of our stress. Anti-anxiety and anti-depressant meds do make a difference. So, does a change in our diet. I started eating more protein, especially for breakfast, to increase my energy level. Carrying extra weight around is stressful for our bodies also.

12. **Protect your emotions.**
Don't watch too much news on TV; read the newspaper instead — if they're still being printed. Don't let movies or books "yank" your emotions. Go for positive,

relaxing, and light content. Best of all, find comfort in reading God's Word—especially His promises.

13. **Get back to nature. Get a pet.** We live about three or four miles from the ocean. Driving there and walking along the water's edge is like taking a mini vacation. But if I sit home, I miss it and the relaxation/enjoyment that it brings. Take a walk. Go fishing.

When we had our dog, Hildy, I'd put her on my lap and pet her. It's documented proof that animals are good for our blood pressure.

14. **Connect with God.**
Spend time in meditation and prayer every day. We are spiritual beings in these physical bodies. To find release from stress, balance in your life, and peace in your heart, spending time with God is the key.

Have a regular place. I sit on my swivel rocker, in our living room, and put my feet up on the stool.

Have a regular time. I eat breakfast, read the newspaper, and meet God— in the morning.

Have a routine. I pray with a daily list and read and highlight my Bible. (The Bible is our only accurate guide—it's God's direct message to us. Other books are good, but don't neglect the main one.)

Keep a spiritual journal. I record some Scripture and other thoughts from devotional books each day.

**Imagine God inviting you
to hand over your tensions and worries to Him.
Doesn't that sound good?**

**He's willing.
Are you?**

It's been over 15 years since my ambulance ride when my battle with stress began in earnest. I still carry its effects in my body, and it swings back into full bloom with the least amount of coaxing. But I have learned when and where to use the stress reducers chronicled above.

I also know that this event was also my "polio crash," and it intensified my post-polio symptoms. (Later in this book you'll read more about how I struggled and am still coping with that chapter (polio) in my life.)

But no matter the cause of your stress, I highly recommend that you start with God. Connecting with God will improve more than your stress.

II Corinthians 1:9,10 LB says, *...we saw how powerless we were to help ourselves; but that was good, for then we put everything into the hands of God...And He did help us...and we expect Him to do it again and again.*

Suggested Reading
The Anxiety Cure by Dr. Archibald D. Hart
The Overload Syndrome by Dr. Richard Swenson

Be patient with elderly people
who rehearse their aches and pains.
You'll be playing your own "organ" recital someday.

Excerpt from
A King-Size Bed, A Silk Tree & A Fry Pan

A Cup of Cold Water

And whoever . . . gives to one of these little ones even a cup of cold water . . .   Matt. 10:42 (ESV)

Wouldn't it be nice to serve God by handing out glasses of cold water? That's a job I could handle, or at least I used to think so, until God placed our family in Africa — five degrees above the steamy equator — for two years. There a cold drink was a precious commodity.

My refrigerator was apartment-size, the ice cube trays numbered only two, and foods not normally refrigerated in the United States had to be in the tropics. My fridge was full. There was room for only two half-gallon containers of water. I was very careful to keep them filled. (Remember that in the tropics water runs warm from the faucet.)

People would ask us for a drink of water knowing that we had a refrigerator — that meant *cold* water. The lady who came with fruit would want a drink. The boys who picked coconuts, the young men who worked for the mission, the men doing repair work, and some days a truck of four or five men from the port would all want a drink.

There I would be—suppertime, and no cold water for my family. Oh, how I came to dread handing out cups of cold water. The price of paper cups was prohibitive. Each drink given out also meant another glass to wash. If I sent out one glass for three people to use, that would be an insult. At their own homes, from their own people, it was accepted; but from Westerners it would never do.

I came to hate handing out drinks of cold water. I tried not to be available when I suspected a request was about to come to my door, or I had my house-help hand out the drinks.

A drink of cold water had become worth gold to me. Finally, God showed me that my attitude was ruining any testimony that I could have gained by cheerfully giving cups of cold water. Even when my family had to drink luke-warm Kool-Aid, I tried to smile.

My thoughts about an "easy way" to serve God returned. How mistaken I had been. Don't ever wish you could do something easier for God. You just might end up on the other side of the ocean and find out that the job really isn't all that simple.

Written November 1989

Do you want to read more?

Order the entire book, *A King-Size Bed, A Silk Tree & A Fry Pan*, at Amazon.com or an online bookstore.

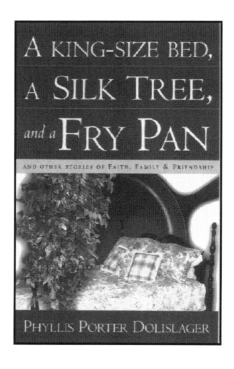

Believing that the wisdom acquired in a lifetime is as much a part of a family's legacy as are all of its material possession, Phyllis Dolislager uses stories from her family's lives to illustrate what's truly important to her and her husband.

Stories of trusting God, helping others, as well as struggles faced, make this book meaningful not only to her family but to all who read it.

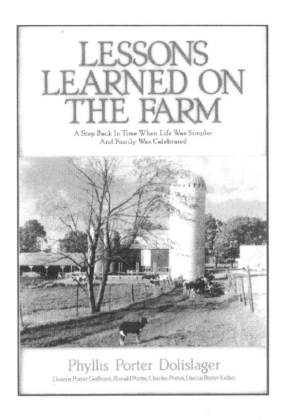

Synopsis of book

This family memoir is set in rural Michigan, where the family farm provides the backdrop for hard work, innovation and overcoming tragedy. Filled with nostalgia from the 50s and 60s, including over 70 photos and a farm diary from 1963, enjoy a step back in time when life was simpler, and family was celebrated. A two-room country school, a country church, and a mother who was a true partner, all provided the perfect training ground for developing discipline, integrity, work ethic, and love of God.

Excerpts from
Lessons Learned on the Farm

Chapter 3
Hard Work and Innovation

Farming, some people say, is the same as gambling. When you plant the seed, you gamble on the price at harvest time. You gamble on whether or not there will be enough sunshine to bring your crop to maturity. You gamble on whether there will be enough rain. You gamble that you'll be able to keep your equipment in good repair, and whether you'll be able to hire the extra hands that will be needed for the harvest.

Basically, it's you against Mother Nature. In the spring we prayed for the snow to dissipate and the fields to dry out enough to plant. The day after we finished planting, we prayed for rain, so the seed would germinate. When we applied Atrazine to the corn, we wanted rain to get it into the soil, and on and on it went.

We wanted rain, and then we didn't want rain— especially if we had a hay crop to bring in. In the fall, the rain would be good for the winter wheat, but interfered with harvesting the corn. And we wanted the corn harvested by Thanksgiving.

The only months that we were free from this weather worry were December through March. Then the cycle would begin all over. It was a topic that consumed us:

the weather. Even if there was hay ready to bale and rain predicted for Monday, we must add that Dad never worked on Sundays,

On a hot day in June as we brought in the first cutting of hay, Dad would say, "This weather is perfect." None of us agreed, but we didn't say a word. Dad would also say that his father or grandfather used to say, "Dry weather — everyone eats; wet weather--everyone looks for something to eat," and "Dry weather you worry to death; wet weather you starve to death."

On a hot, steamy day in July, he would say, "Today you can hear the corn grow." Grandpa Porter used to say that the corn crop should be knee-high by the Fourth of July and shoulder-high by August. But with the hybrid seed that we used, that saying became outdated. We wanted our corn to be shoulder-high by the Fourth of July and to have tassels by August.

Chapter 4
Heartbeat of the Farm Family

We drank milk with all of our meals. Mother kept it in various sized glass jars in our refrigerator. The tops of all the jars would be thick with the cream that would rise to the top. None of us liked the thick taste of cream. We'd always stick a knife into the bottle and "stir up the milk" before pouring it. We drank "raw" milk — it wasn't pasteurized. City folks thought that was unhealthy and unwise, and we thought that "city" milk tasted horrid and refused to drink it. Neighbors were shocked to hear that Mother fed Chuck and Dar "raw" milk mixed with Karo syrup. She'd bring the milk to a boil, add the syrup, and that was their formula.

Chapter 5
Country School and Beyond

It was a sure sign of spring when we started riding our bikes to school again. The roads were gravel — sometimes soft, sometimes bumpy with ruts. They didn't get paved until Dar's last year at Courtland Center. We had to be skillful and careful. Our bikes didn't have gears, and their balloon tires had no special treads. All of our bikes did have metal baskets. We carried our lunches in them and anything else we wanted at school. More than one glass-lined thermos was broken as the bike rider crashed on the way to or from school.

Chapter 6
Twice a Day — 365 Days a Year

Knowing that the cows were waiting to be milked didn't make getting out of bed easy. The chore faced us twice a day, every day of the year, without exception. But by the time we got out the door of the house and were walking on the path toward the barn, we were resigned. We'd open the gate into the barnyard and push the red barn door along its sliding track to our left. If it was cold, the warmth from the cows' bodies would immediately strike us. Dad always had a wide-awake greeting for us.

To him, this was the best place in the world to be. We never saw him begrudge milking cows.

As we'd stand in the open barn door and face south, we could look across the barnyard, down the lane, past the pasture and crops to the woods. Our workplaces and results of our labor were always in sight. Then we'd turn around and go into the barn where milking the cows was our immediate concern. Chuck says it was some of the best times he spent with Dad. The radio would be tuned to WOOD-AM where Buck Barry at 5 AM and Bruce Grant at 6 AM would accompany us as we did our chores and watched the sun rise over the pasture.

* * *

Once when Chuck was washing a cow's udder, she started kicking him. Dad had taught us to put our shoulder into the cow and push her over. But this cow continued her kicking. It was so bad; Chuck had to finally crawl out by the cow's head instead of backing out. We never saw Dad beat our cows, but he was so upset with this cow that he sold her for beef the very next day.

* * *

Prince was bought for Chuck and Dar, but he became a horse that Dad actually liked. Dad bought him at

Ravenna at the auction. He was black and white and sold with his saddle on. Imagine Dad's surprise when he took the saddle off to see the biggest sway back ever! Then he understood why the saddle had been included. Dad would ride Prince and even used him to herd the cows.

Do you want to read more?

Order the entire book, *Lessons Learned on the Farm*, at Amazon.com or at an online bookstore.

Who Hit the "Down" Button?

Feelings about a chronic illness

I always knew that I was living on an elevator.
I remember stopping at certain floors.
Some I anticipated — like teaching
      and giving my Writing Workshops.
I wanted to stay and browse there all day.
A couple of times I'd inadvertently, I think,
      gotten off at the wrong floor.
What in the world was I doing participating in a mock
      jury?
      Testing mouthwashes?
      Handing out food samples?
Oh yes; now I remember.
I was between jobs, and any extra money was
      appreciated.

Some of the floors held more for me than others, and I always did enjoy finding specials. The linens and dishes fascinated me. I loved them all.

And then there was the shoe floor. I visited there often. Having a size 7 right foot, and a size 10 left foot, shoe shopping became a challenge, until . . . I found Jean, in Minnesota (now deceased), who had the exact opposite size feet as mine.

As the elevator continued to climb ever upward, reaching new floors,

I added another degree behind my name.
We lived . . . in Africa . . . for two years!
Then we moved to Florida.

And all too soon we were traveling again . . . to our sons'
weddings . . . then to their children's
baptisms.
    But . . . somewhere . . . in the busyness . . .
        I lost track of which floor I was on . . .
           and what I was looking for . . ..

In fact, I woke up one day, and the elevator, my trusty
source of motivation and transport was . . .
      going . . .
        down!

What happened?
Who changed directions on me?
I'm not used to this downward motion.
I DON'T LIKE IT.
Oh God, did I do something wrong?
What is this?
I'm not working . . . or . . . shopping . . . or even sleeping.
Where's my social life? I miss it.
And what is this pain all about?
When did this all happen?
How did I change directions without even knowing it?

The change was gradual, for a while.
The tension sneaked up and climbed onto my shoulders.

I woke up with chest pains.
I brought my work home and thought about it 24/7.
Even on vacation . . ..
I will never forget sitting in the Sheraton Hotel,
        overlooking Niagara Falls, reading a Federal
        RFP (request for proposal).

OK, so I did stop and stay too long on some floors,
but I don't remember the elevator changing directions.
I just remember the fatigue, lying on the couch after
work, and wishing for a massage every day.

I now know that I changed directions about 2001.
I also know that I can't do today what I could do a year
        ago . . . or even six months ago.
Has the speed of the down elevator accelerated?
More than once the thought crossed my mind
        that I wished that I had a wheelchair
        because walking had become such an effort.
I also know that my dream of going to Paris won't
        happen—unless it's in a wheelchair.

Ron does the grocery shopping, or I have them
        delivered.
I can shop for 10 items or less, but the last time I shopped
for a week's worth of groceries, I had fatigue and muscle
weakness for two days.

And just last week,
I had to have someone start cleaning house for me.

If I need clothes, I can go to only one store, and I hope and pray that they'll have what I need, in my size, at my price.

I never thought that my shopping genes would be affected.

POLIO

Yes, it's affected my life since I was 18 months old.
I've spent 60+ years working around it . . . overcoming
it . . . trying to forget it.

BUT it's become a guest who's outstayed its welcome.
It's hard to know what to do with it . . . and its
      consequences.

Now we use a new name: POST-POLIO SYNDROME,
      or the Late Effects of Polio.
1.3 million of us in the U.S. have it.
One friend calls it, "The gift that keeps on giving."
Like it or not, we have no choice but to accept its "gifts"
      of knee braces, canes, pain medications,
      wheelchairs or scooters,
      and our loss of freedom and social activities.

There are days that I literally grieve for my former life
*   on the "up" elevator.*

The prognosis, you ask?
There's little chance for improvement; the odds are
      heavily weighted in the direction of a
      downward spiral.
BUT my mind continues to spin out of control with ideas
      that my body can no longer accomplish.
This might be my biggest frustration.
YET if my mind were to lose its creativity, I'd be
      devastated.

So, in the long run, I do have a lot to be thankful for.

Then there's my faith.
If I didn't firmly believe that God is the Blessed Controller of all things, I would be devastated.
In his book, *The Purpose Driven Life*, Rick Warren says,
> "Your circumstances are temporary,
> but your character will last forever."

Personally, I think that using "wheelchair" in the same sentence with my own name, is building as much character as I could ever wish for.

Believing that good can come out of bad,
> I'm waiting . . .
> not anticipating . . . but waiting . . .
> to see how this "character thing" plays out.

ᎤᏍᎡ ᎡᏬᎦ ᎤᏍᎡ

1. When was it official that you had a chronic illness or disability?
2. What was your first reaction?
3. How long did it take for you to come to acceptance?
4. Have you come to acceptance?

Do you know someone with a chronic illness or disability who would benefit from reading this?

For 21 more similar articles and questions,

> *Who Hit the Down Button,*
> Life with a Chronic Illness or Disability

is available at Amazon.com or other online booksellers.

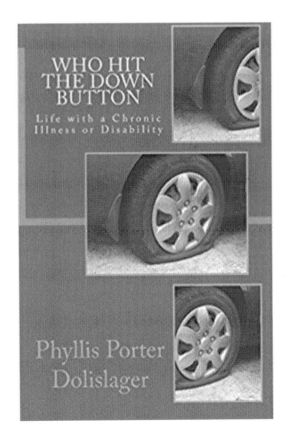

*What Is Post-Polio Syndrome?

Post-Polio Syndrome (PPS), The Late Effects of Poliomyelitis are the unexpected and often disabling symptoms -- overwhelming fatigue, muscle weakness, muscle and joint pain, sleep disorders, heightened sensitivity to anesthesia, cold and pain, as well as difficulty swallowing and breathing -- that occur about 35 years after the poliovirus attack in 75% of paralytic and 40% of "non-paralytic" polio survivors.[1]

What Causes PPS?

PPS is caused by decades of "overuse abuse." The poliovirus damaged 95% of the brain stem and spinal cord motor neurons, killing at least 50%. Virtually every muscle in the body was affected by polio, as were brain-activating neurons that keep the brain awake and focus attention. Although damaged, the remaining neurons compensated by sending out "sprouts," like extra telephone lines, to activate muscles that were orphaned when their neurons were killed. These over-sprouted, poliovirus-damaged neurons are now failing and dying from overuse, causing muscle weakness and fatigue. Overuse of weakened muscles causes muscle and joint pain, as well as difficulty with breathing and swallowing.[2]

For more information about the cause and treatment of PPS go to
[1,2]www.postpolioinfo.com

Rules for Smoking . . . for Five-Year Olds
A little humor along the way

The rules we impose on our children have everything to do with current, cultural taboos. It's only after 30+ years have passed that I can laugh at one rule I set down for Fred, our older son. At the age of five, I told him that he could only smoke in his bedroom — not in any other room of the house, or outside.

Smoke? At the age of five? Those were the days of candy cigarettes. They came in a cardboard box, almost the size of a regular pack of cigarettes. They were white, sweet sticks with one end painted red to simulate realness.

If an adult held a candy cigarette, it looked real. But when a child held one, any good mother was ready to faint dead away or take some action she might regret the rest of her life.

Unfortunately, depending on your point of view, I decided that I should consider not only the immediate consequences of smoking candy cigarettes, but the future ones as well.

Psychology tells us that what we cannot have or are banned from has a good chance of becoming a future goal. So, I had to decide: was it better to give in to his childish desire for candy cigarettes or to deny his current urge and maybe face a child who would become an adult smoker?

To me this was a weighty issue, and I didn't debate it very long before I decided that candy cigarettes were definitely the lesser of two evils.

A couple of days later, my mother, Fred's Grandma Porter, stopped by for a visit just as Fred had "lit up" a cigarette. She couldn't believe her eyes! She was upset. She cried. Finally, in desperation, she offered Fred money to go buy a WHOLE BAG of candy if he'd "quit smoking."

Fred did not give her a quick response. His five-year-old brain seemed to weigh the decision heavily before giving his answer. Finally, he told Grandma Porter, "No." He wanted to keep smoking his candy cigarettes.

That response confirmed my fears: I had a problem smoker on my hands! After Grandma left, I knew I had to find a compromise. I didn't want Fred's "smoking" to "cause others to stumble" or Grandma to become hysterical every time she saw a cigarette in Fred's mouth.

The solution? Fred had to confine his "smoking" to his bedroom. Without an audience, his habit quickly became history.

Did my 70's psychology work?

> Yes, Fred does not smoke cigarettes today.

Did my 70's psychology fail?

> Yes, Fred prefers cigars today.
> Maybe if Fred had had some chocolate cigars . . .

Who's in Control?

My first experience in a wheelchair almost ended in divorce court. Knowing that I'd never make it on my polio feet for three days at the National Booksellers Convention, I gave in and got a manual wheelchair. My husband Ron, bless his heart, willingly agreed to be my pusher.

Immediately we found an obstacle just getting from our hotel to the Orlando Convention Center next door. Fortunately, I could get out of the chair as he carried it up/down five or six steps. We figured out where the elevators were in the Convention Center, despaired that there was so much carpeting, but how were we to know that the popular book *Men Are from Mars and Women Are from Venus* was going to be our main problem?

I had taken seven copies of my latest book proposal with me. Selling one's self and one's book idea in three to five sentences is a precise skill. Timing is key. Imagine having made a great presentation, followed by a positive response, handing over the proposal, saying good-bye, but not moving. And having this happen more than once.

I knew right then and there that I needed my own power. This person had to regain some control over her life. Three days in a manual chair—even with the world's best husband standing behind me and pushing me — was all it took. Decision time was here. But what was the solution?

Then we attended the Abilities Expos in Ft. Lauderdale, Florida and Doug of T.D. Medical introduced us to the EZ Power Chair. I wanted one!

* * *

My first trip to the mall with my power chair will forever be burned into my memory. With my sore right arm (I now know that it's a torn rotator cuff.), there was no way I could lift the chair into and out of the car's trunk by myself. Even though the power chair breaks down into three pieces, the heaviest piece is 29 pounds. My dear friend Evie Opitz was visiting and offered to accompany me on my trip to the mall — my first in three years!!! This was going to be a BIG day.

First, we practiced taking the chair apart, putting it into the trunk, and then taking it out and assembling it again. With Ron and Evie's husband, Al, looking on and offering all kinds of verbal instruction, we hoped that we had it firmly in mind, and off to the mall we went.

We parked at the Sears end of the mall, opened the trunk, and together unloaded the parts of the chair, and assembled it. Then I sat in my chair, and we were off to do our shopping.

But alas, getting through the door into Sears wasn't all that easy. It felt like I had to literally go left, go right, go left, and go right until I wiggled my way into the store. It was with a sigh of relief that we finally began my long-awaited, shopping trip.

What looked like "forward march" immediately became a "mine field." As I passed by a round table with a long, blue skirt, it started shedding small boxes of jewelry. They tumbled off falling randomly about me. I stopped, but I couldn't see that I owned any responsibility. I started to move, more boxes tumbled. I stopped, the boxes stopped. I'd start, and they'd throw themselves to the ground again.

Needing some assurance that I wasn't at fault, I looked around for Evie. There she was, immediately behind me, bent over in laughter. I mean, she was holding her sides she was laughing so hard. Catching my eye, she said, "Stop. Turn it off." As I realized that I hadn't been able to even start shopping without causing destruction, I was ready to cry. But there was my usually dignified friend laughing her head off. And that calmed me down, and I was able to see the humor.

As she untangled the hem of the table skirt from my chair's axle, she continued to laugh. So instead of retreating to the car, I continued our "forward march" past numerous brightly colored tables with skirts holding more boxes of jewelry.

Three hours later, with our purchases stuffed into the storage area under my seat, we headed back through Sears to the car. This time we by-passed the skirted, "mine field," and I even made it through the doorway without bouncing back and forth, hitting its sides.

As we disassembled the wheelchair and placed its parts, plus our packages, into the car's trunk, it was with a true sense of accomplishment and a smile on my face that I, the proud owner of a power chair, headed home.

We Are Polio Survivors

Long before we'd heard of body types,
personality profiles, or right brain/left brain—
We finished what we'd begun and always did our best.
Work ethic. We had it. We were survivors.

As we grew and matured, no one needed
to encourage us.
We gave ourselves more pressure
than we could handle.
We were Type A: hard-driving, time-conscious,
overachieving perfectionists.

We personified self-esteem. We knew all about drive.
We were survivors.

And then post-polio syndrome reared its ugly head,
and we tasted our first loss of confidence
since contracting polio.

And it was a major loss: our health, our bodies.
We were letting ourselves down; we were failing.
This was a new experience for us.
We didn't know how to handle it.
We were survivors.

Embrace an assistive device? Take a nap?
Ask for help?
What ridiculous mirage was this!
We were the survivors—not the losers.

It's taken us time to accept our new limitations.
We'd rather die in battle . . . than give up.

But one by one our Type A personalities have shifted to
the opposite side of our brains, and we decided that if
we were going to have a life . . . we needed to embrace
our naps, use our assistive devices,
and once again become survivors.

Now we buy mini vans to transport our electric
scooters and wheelchairs. We take vacations on
accommodating cruise lines. And reluctantly, we admit
how stubborn we'd been not to accept the help that had
been available to us years earlier.

We're still Type A.
Our minds haven't stopped working.
But now we're educating our younger doctors
about post-polio
and striving for enforcement of the [1]ADA.
Thank God, we still have a job to do!
We are survivors.

[1] Americans with Disabilities Act

Written October 3 and 4, 2003
Inspired by Jody Taylor who said,
"I should have gotten this powered wheelchair two years ago."

Special People

I think there will be a special place in heaven
for caregivers.

You who have loaded wheelchairs into cars or vans,
or cut up food and gently placed
it into your mate's mouth,
or emptied bladder bags or positioned sleep machines.
There must be a special place for you.

Have you stood in line to buy take-out?
or stopped for groceries on your way home from work?
There's a special place in our hearts for you.

Have you held the hand of your ill, loved-one and
reminded them of why you chose to marry him/her
in the first place?
And then added the reasons
why you'd do it all over again?
There's a special reward in heaven for you.

You may think that no one knows,
and no one cares or understands,
but you're wrong, my friend.

Remember, Scripture says,
Show mercy and compassion to one another.
Zechariah 7:9 (NKJV)

This week hold your head a little higher and
place a smile on your face.
For someone sees your acts of kindness
He cares, and He remembers.

Written October 27, 2003
After dinner with post-polio friends

TENNESSEE POETRY

Haute Couture in East Tennessee
The dogwoods modeled their pink and white dresses;
The red buds flaunted their new spring apparel.
While the tulips paraded in multicolored skirts
And sprightly strutted from yard to yard.

Forsythia posed on the hills and the roadsides
Where the daffodils flirtingly waved to us.
One should drive slowly when viewing God's runway
That weaves around the mountain and into town.

April 2007

Their Favorite Time of Year

With smiles on their faces
the trees swayed ever so smugly.
For they were proudly wearing
their new, vivid-green skirts.

Through the long winter months
they'd been forced to wear pants —
dark brown pants and black pants.
No wonder spring is their favorite season.

May/07

Contentment

The mountains don't complain;
They continue to pose for us.
No matter the season,
no matter the weather.

But I wonder . . .
Do they ever wish that they could jump rope
or skip from cove to cove calling,
"You're it" to their nearest neighbor?

Or are they content to sit
with their hands folded in their lap--
an inspiration to all mankind
who come to gaze on their majesty?

Their silent beauty stretches before us
proclaiming the awesomeness of God.
Oh, that you and I could be more like
the non-complaining mountains.

5/2007

Mountain Drama

Spring and summer schedule shows
for which the mountains quit shaving.
Their leafy green beards grow and
begin to hide their crag-like faces.

They look forward to these performances.
It's as if they put on disguises
and can tour incognito
as one looks almost like the other.

But each year, autumn
quietly sneaks up on them.
First their leafy costume changes color,
and then it disappears all together.

When winter arrives,
their true identity is revealed
as their stoic countenance
is dramatically unmasked.

Without the changing of the seasons,
we wouldn't have seats for this annual drama.
God's glorious spectacle
receives rave reviews each year.

7/17/07

I Never Burned My Bra, but . . .

I never burned my bra, but I did refuse to use/say the word "obey" in my marriage vows. (The pastor changed the word to "cherish," the same one that Ron said in his vows.) It was the 60's, and some of us women decided to transform the status quo. We women wanted to do what men were doing — and to be paid the same rate.

The main careers for women, who were lucky enough to go to college, were teaching and nursing. In 1963, the year I graduated from college, only 39% of college graduates were female.[1] My sister-in-law, a pediatrician, was turned down by several medical schools. The prevailing thought at the time was that only men could make it as a doctor — women would be asking for time off to have babies, etc. Thank goodness since that time the prevailing thought has changed! According to the AMA, since the 1970s, the proportion of female medical students has risen greatly although their average salaries still are not equal.[2]

Early in my teaching career, I quit a job as a writing adjunct at a local university in Michigan. A full-time position opened up, and of course, that's what every adjunct was hoping would come her way. But . . . it was

[1, 2] National Center for Education Statistics

given to a man – a man with no experience teaching that course. And I had taught the very same course the previous semester – my job review was fine. The administration was shocked that I quit – it really rocked their boat. Hopefully it made them think long and hard the next time they were faced with a similar situation.

Later at a prep school in Florida where I had been hired to teach speech and drama, I learned that a male teacher was being paid an extra stipend to coach junior varsity golf. Previously when I had directed plays and coached debate, I had received extra pay too. But this school had led me to believe that those extra-curricular activities were part of my job – no extra compensation. When I discovered that my colleague was "being paid to play golf," I spoke up, and I received an extra stipend also. But why had that happened in the first place?

Women are a powerful force in the workplace today because years ago some of us went out on a limb to demand equal rights and equal pay. I think our efforts have been as significant as the women's suffrage movement was in the early 1900's. And the job is not done – probably never will be. But we're no longer viewed as the "weaker" sex. We've set our sights high, and we've gotten other women to "look up" too.

Years later, when I was Program Director for Gold Coast Community Services, federal money was made available for teaching about teen pregnancy and STD prevention in the high schools in the U.S. I wrote and won one of the first federally funded grant proposals. I hired an equal number of guys and gals for teaching and paid them all the same rate. My staff had a profound influence on the students in our county. The rate of teen pregnancies started to decline.

Looking back on my life, the first, big factor that shaped me into the independent woman that I am today . . . was my father. I am amazed that he was ahead of his times, in his goals for me — a *daughter*. I grew up in the 50's and 60's when most families were preparing their *sons* for the future.

However, it was always assumed that *I* would go to college. There was never any question. It wasn't easy for a farmer to send his daughter to college, but it happened. Extra steers were raised, and a lot of prayers were sent heavenward. Even choosing a Christian college, Taylor University, for my first two years was O.K. with him.

I enjoy going back and mulling over the things my father taught me. We'd sit at the kitchen table when he paid the bills once a month, and he'd have me do the actual check writing. What a way for me to learn about all the bills that our family faced. He also taught me how to do income taxes. When I married, it was a turnabout for me to teach my husband how to figure the taxes.

My father was truly a man ahead of his times. Not only was he a successful farmer, but a man who knew how to prepare a daughter for more than she could have ever expected would come her way. Once we went to a cattle auction to purchase a heifer for me to show at the 4-H Fair. He made me do my own bidding . . . helpful in teaching me independence, and that I could do anything I set my mind to.

After I graduated from college, I bought a new car, a 1963 Dodge Dart. A year later, I was again looking at cars, and with my father's encouragement I upgraded (when upgraded wasn't even a word) to a white convertible with blue interior and a blue roof. I'm so glad that he encouraged me to follow my dreams! Even today, I'm the one who "buys" the cars for our family.

What a legacy he gave me! Live your dreams. Don't limit your horizons because you're a woman. And most of all, he taught me to always seek God's will. I salute my father, Darcy Erwin Porter, a man ahead of his time when it came to preparing a daughter to be independent.

All of these life lessons are the source of any empowerment and independence that I possess. What more could an independent woman need or want?

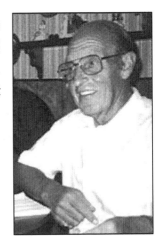

What Happened to Church 101?

We used to go to church and be handed a bulletin with an outline for the sermon, and all the announcements for the week. Then would follow some traditional music and a collection plate was passed by deacons wearing suit coats and ties. A special announcement might bring different people to the microphone.

By the time the sermon was to start, we'd be encouraged to get out our fill-in-the-blanks sermon outline to make sure we GOT the three points. And if one happened to daydream, he/she could always look at the outline held by the person on his/her left or right and belatedly fill in the blanks.

Church 101 — freshman level — everyone got it. Everyone passed. In fact, the answers were on the screen at the front. No adult, teen or child was left behind.

This routine was so predictable that one could place a bet on the actual sequence with a 97% odds of winning. Once we got home, we would trash the sermon outline and check *Church* off our Sunday To-Do List.

Then we found Maryville Vineyard Church, and our brains felt like we'd accidentally gotten into Church 495. What's happening here? Is this what we signed up for? Thinking . . . did I really hear THAT? What's with this music? Be quiet and meditate on Scripture on the big screen. Stand up and hear the guitars, keyboard, and even a drum set sound out. And sometimes there'd be a lady with a violin or a man with a harmonica. There were strange words, yet modern and stranger yet tunes. Is that what they call melody now-a-days? OK. We needed to upgrade our repertoire of church/Christian music.

Next there might be some familiar words sung in a revved-up way — getting us ready for communion. Then comes some exercise, walking to a communion station — one was even gluten free — and then the memory challenge: where was I sitting? Reflection time? Oh, yes. *Thank you, Lord. So glad to do this every Sunday. Really . . . sincerely. We like this . . . a lot!*

The announcements vary from Pastor Sharon or some other staff person like Brooks Coker, who gives them with a bit of humor or a mention of the Vol's football game. Succinct, to the point, often on the big screen. And they have The Box . . . no passing . . . of anything. Just put IT in on your way out. And no one stands at the door to remind you. You're on your own here too. Or you can give online or text it to 97000. Definitely NOT Church 101, and we *definitely* like it.

But the pastor . . . Pastor Aaron McCarter . . . hold onto your seat! He's a tall dude . . . cowboy? Or is it just the jeans? He sits down in front of his iPad and proceeds to talk to us, after showing us shocking images like Jesus with His lips censored! on that big screen. And he likes using props: trying to hit the sound booth man, John Conley, with nerf darts to make his point.

And the sermon . . . we listen . . . hard . . . we take notes. And Church 495 — *senior level* — really begins. It's like a lecture. You're on your own to get the points. Oh, he tells us, once, but it's way above Church 101. Church 495 isn't for sissies. It's ADULTS-ONLY. And Sunday after Sunday we're stretched, poked, prodded to learn more — to understand more about God.

Maryville Vineyard Church doesn't censor Jesus. No. We leave with new insights/understanding of Scripture that we've previously read and taken at face value. "It forces its way in. It's disruptive and it changes everything. It's simple, but not easy," says Pastor Aaron. "This message of Jesus requires us to take ourselves out of the center of our lives, and to put God on center stage. We exist to applaud God; we are to stop performing."

And while these concepts buzz around our head, the tall dude in the jeans talks passionately, quietly as if this were as routine as singing "Jesus Loves Me". He wants people from Church 101 to understand Church 495. And we do . . . we do remember handing the stage and the leading role to God. But our minds have been stretched. Maybe this is really a graduate-level course.

And Pastor Aaron is right—it doesn't count what we've already done. It's all about NOW. Who's on center stage in my life *now . . . today . . . in East Tennessee?*

And I feel the rush. I've learned something. I understand Scripture like never before. Maybe I do belong in Church 495. I don't even want to think about Church 101. That was a hundred years ago, wasn't it?

--originally written 2012, revised 2019

Reading . . . and Writing

Reading was a lifeline for me.
It's how my mother kept me lying flat in bed
when I had polio as a two-year old.
She read to me.

I learned all the nursery rhymes
and all the fairy tales.
When I finished kindergarten,
I was promoted to second grade.

Then the book mobile came
to our country school,
and I was reading for myself.
I devoured the Little House
on the Prairie books.

Our family subscribed to the daily newspaper,
and I eagerly anticipated each new installment
of Uncle Wiggly.

In church, I shifted gears,
and I learned to read the Bible.

Then it was on to high school
and more intense reading and writing.

I worked as an aide in the high school library.
Would I ever have made it to college
without my love of reading that had been so
finely developed?

When I became a high school teacher,
I read love letters from my future husband,
Ron.
I knew I was going to marry him
at our first meeting,
but I fell in love with him
from reading his letters.

And the cycle of reading continued
as we read to our sons, Fred and Tom.

Now, I not only continue to read,
but I also write.
Perhaps it's only fitting that my most-read
book is
Lessons Learned on the Farm
where reading began for me.

Ferris Wheels & Merry-Go-Rounds
Counterculture Shock

From the Ferris wheel to the merry-go-round in twelve hours . . . we could do that. It should be simple. We'd lived in the land of merry-go-rounds all our lives, and only the last two years had we taken up residence in the country of Ferris wheels.

Yes, we'd been told stories about the land of Ferris wheels before our arrival. We thought we could make that continuous, big circle up-high-into-the-air and then down-to-the-ground again. We had people praying for us, so that when it stopped at the top and rocked (poisonous snakes, military coups, malaria) we wouldn't be afraid, but would trust God.

Our transition to Ferris wheels did go fairly well. We learned to dicker over prices for vegetables, to stand in line at the post office for an hour, to light the kerosene lanterns when the lights went out, and to say an extra prayer when we discovered that our boys had eaten a bird which had been cooked — feathers and all — over an open fire.

Life in the land of Ferris wheels became almost routine for us. We could go up . . . come down . . . and even enjoy the ride. But after two years, it was time to return to the land of the merry-go-rounds. We'd ridden them since childhood and eagerly anticipated joining our relatives and friends on that great ride.

We returned to be greeted and helped up on the ride. We hung on tightly and tried to enjoy ourselves. But the old fun wasn't there. The merry-go-round was suddenly complicated. It went around in circles . . . and the horses . . . went up and down . . . all at the same time. Frankly, we felt dizzy — but we attempted to keep smiles pasted on our faces.

All too soon, our friends and relatives, assuming that we knew all about life in the land of merry-go-rounds, left us on our own. Little did they, or we, know that occasionally they should have been sitting behind us, helping us hang on. Of course, we *had* been masters at this before.   We needed to buy a "horse." In the land of Ferris wheels, there were only three places to shop for a "horse," but now we were faced with dozens of "horse" dealerships, "horses" parked in driveways with FOR SALE signs, and friends with "horses" for sale. Everyone in the land of merry-go-rounds owns one or two "horses." They also freely give advice about choices and prices.

When shopping for bread in grocery stores, we had to *choose* from countless brands, and at the same time not pay too much. This myriad of choices continued for each item on our grocery list. Checking out posed more difficulties. The clerk almost assailed me because I didn't have any coupons clenched in my hand to offer her. And, I'd forgotten how to write checks. It took me much too long by the clerk's standards. (In the land of Ferris wheels, we'd used only cash. But this land of merry-go-rounds uses little cash.)

The shopping malls posed more problems. They were . . . big . . . clean . . . so much merchandise . . . I was overwhelmed. We had to leave soon after our first visit as I became so nauseous I thought I'd vomit. We were also reminded that in the land of merry-go-rounds, it wasn't right to just "buy" underwear, but it should also be "on sale." This meant more time shopping in the "threatening" stores. This was especially true for people who had just been to the land of Ferris wheels — others watched closely to make sure that our spending habits were conservative.

Gradually we transitioned back to the merry-go-round. We bought our own "horses." Ron took his to work, and I had one too. (That's the way in this land.) We learned not to buy gas at the first station we passed--each station might have a different price. We learned to save coupons. We learned to shop at garage sales. (Not too unlike the open-air markets we had become accustomed to in the land of Ferris wheels.)

Little by little that going-around-in-circles-while-going-up-and-down became routine for us. Good ole merry-go-rounds. Yes, we did miss you.

This article was written in 1980
about our return to life in the U.S.
after two years in Liberia, West Africa.

Talk to Strangers: Say Hello

An orange T-shirt, two people reading from the same book, and the last episode of the Sopranos. What could these three things possibly have in common?

My husband and I were enjoying the beach one day — the sound of the waves breaking, the blue sky and the warm sunshine. Out of the corner of my eye I saw another couple coming down to the beach. Later I noticed that they had placed their chaise lounges about as close to one another as possible, and they appeared to be reading. But what really caught my attention was that there was only one book between the two of them.

After glancing their way a couple of times to confirm my suspicion, I had to get up and ask, "Are you guys reading the same book?" Their response was, "Yes, we do it all the time."

There went the whole theory of "Men are from Mars, and Women are from Venus." This man and woman were from the same planet! But I soon found out that they weren't from the U.S. They were from Germany.

This fact opened a whole conversation and an urge to get better acquainted. Eventually we spent time together. We showed them some local sights, including an alligator, and helped them reel in their first fish. Later they took us out for dinner as a thank you.

We're hoping to keep in touch. Already they've emailed us some photos from our adventures together. I gave them a book I had written, and I was pleased to hear that they read it — together — on their trip home.

Ready for something a little more eclectic than Palm Beach, we headed to Key West for a few days. And yes, our lives were immediately pulled out of the routine. We arrived on Fat Tuesday and the bizarre residents of Key West were out en mass. Add to that the one or two thousand chickens that roam the streets, and the large number of tourists, and the festival was 'a happenin'.

A couple of mornings later, as we sat in the courtyard of our bed and breakfast, a gal walked out of her room wearing an orange T-shirt. And it was a University of Tennessee color of orange. I had to ask, "Are you from Tennessee?" Her response was, "No. I'm from Rockford, Illinois."

I couldn't let that pass. I had to tell her that I grew up near Rockford, Michigan, and my Rockford was named after her Rockford.

Being as gregarious as I am, she inquired about my knee brace. I told her that I was Post-Polio. She replied that she and her husband had two relatives who were also. As I have written about polio quite a lot, I asked if she'd like some of my small books for them.

While explaining the chapter titles, she said, "Stop. My husband needs to hear this." As he walked out, I could tell there was something different about his leg, and of course, I asked.

He shared his story of a car accident, losing his foot, and the effect it had on his professional life as a dentist. In the process, we learned that he wasn't used to sharing his story. This was something new for him.

When he finished telling us his story, I asked him, "How did this make you feel?"

He asked, "Psychologically?" I nodded, yes. He answered, "Great!"

I encouraged him to continue to share his story and to also reach out to younger people to help them cope with similar loses. Later I wrote them both letters with some more suggestions. What a rewarding memory from meeting those two, amazing people.

Back at our condo in Palm Beach, the banter continued between Rudy, a neighbor, and me. I had already learned that he had owned an ice cream shop in New Jersey. I also knew that they made their own ice cream, sauces and fudge. But one day Rudy added a choice morsel to our on-going conversation: the last episode of the Sopranos had been filmed in his shop.

He had my attention. "Wow," I said, "I bet you made a bundle from that!" He replied, "The bigger bundle came from the sale of the T-shirts and mugs after the shooting." Ah, Rudy . . . always a man with one more tidbit of interest.

Later I learned that the first day he and his wife moved to the U.S. from Germany, he put on an apron, and started working behind the counter of a deli. Nine months later, he was managing the deli. And four years after that, he bought the now famous ice cream parlor that seats 100 and has 28 to 30 employees.

Fascinating people all around us—all the time. But on vacation we finally slow down, take time to smell the flowers (or the chickens), and to say hello to a stranger. And look what it brought me: new friends, an opportunity to help someone, and a good story to share with you. Rudy isn't the only one with some interesting tidbits these days!

Angel Does Guard Duty . . . and . . . GPS

It was my first night alone in the rustic cabin in Norris Dam State Park in Tennessee, and I was afraid. Every pinecone that fell on the roof sounded like a brick or a bullet to me. But then I wasn't entirely sure that it came from the surrounding trees; someone with an evil intent might have thrown something.

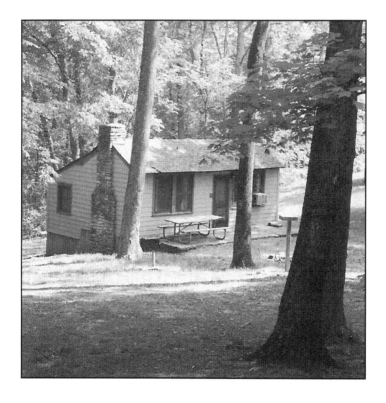

I had reserved this cabin for two and a half weeks to work on a family memoir knowing that "rustic" meant no phone service. But I hadn't planned on strange sounds, animals on the prowl during the night, or a cabin 300 feet away full of men from a construction job. To top it off, the cabin across from me was empty.

"Dear God," I prayed as I lay in bed, "What am I going to do? I can't spend this entire time being tense and afraid. I came here to write — to be productive."

Almost immediately I had this picture in my mind of a large angel, sitting just outside the cabin, on top of the picnic table. He was sitting erect with his arms crossed in front, and he was on full alert/guard duty.

I breathed freely and softly said, "Thank you, God." For the entire two and a half weeks I had no fear: my guardian angel was there, protecting me.

When it was time to pack up and head to the mountains in North Carolina for two more weeks of writing, my old fears returned. But this time I was worried about driving so far on my own, getting lost, or just plain having car trouble.

Once again God sent my guardian angel and made him visible in my mind's eye. You won't believe where he rode the whole trip — on the top of my car — with his arms still folded across his chest — on full alert — looking straight ahead at the road and the on-coming traffic.

What a comforting feeling! What an immediate answer to my prayer! And what fun I have sharing this story of God's provision and protection. In fact, my friend Mimi has said on more than one occasion that she wanted to "borrow my angel." And that's just fine with me.

Dear Friend, what fears are you facing today? Loneliness, misunderstanding, financial problems, guilt, depression, inadequacies, fatigue, lack of appreciation?

Tell them to your Heavenly Father. He truly cares for you and has angels ready to rescue you and guide you.

Do not be afraid of the terrors of the night,
Nor fear the dangers of the day,
For he orders his angels
To protect you wherever you go.

Psalm 91:5, 11 (NLT)

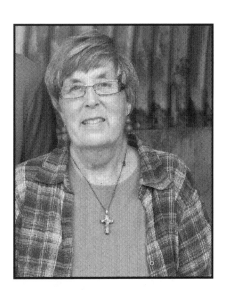

About the Author

Phyllis Dolislager freelances as a writing consultant. For Christmas 2000, Phyllis wrote her Testament, *A King-Size Bed, A Silk Tree & A Fry Plan,* and other stories of Faith, Family & Friends, for her family.

After she wrote her Testament, her Michigan family requested a similar book about the Porter family and growing up on the farm in the 50's and 60's. Consequently, she is the author of the family memoir: *Lessons Learned on the Farm,* A Step Back in Time When Life Was Simpler and Family Was Celebrated.

Miscellaneous . . . The Book, is her 11th book. It's a compilation of poetry, essays, and writings from other family members—including a "secret" hot dog chili sauce recipe. To learn more about her other books visit Amazon.com and other online booksellers.

Made in the
USA
Lexington, KY